Vegan Diet

High Protein Salad Recipes To Suppress Cravings And Achieve Rapid Weight Loss

(Nutritious Suggestions, And Expert Counsel To Encourage A Vegan Lifestyle And Improve Liver Function)

EkkehardBartl

TABLE OF CONTENT

Overview Of The Vegan Diet 1

Basics Of Veganism 6

How To Make The Switch To A Vegan Diet 9

The Breakfast Sandwich 15

Squishy Chocolate Chipcakes 19

Vegan Diet Proven Benefits 21

Crucial Information On Nutrition 26

Salad With Couscous 42

Pancakes With Blueberries 45

How To Eat A Balanced Diet Without Tracking Calories 52

Why Make The Vegan Switch? 63

The Foundations Of High-Protein Vegan Dietary Plans 76

Little Carrot Cakes For Breakfast 80

Breakfast Burrito For Vegans With Tofu Scramble 83

Accepting The Shift: A Guide To Lectin-Free Vegan Transition 97

How To Begin Cooking With Pegans 123

Yummy Vegan Chronosomic Cookbook 129

1. Quinoa Power Bowl 129

CRISPY Baked ZUCCHINI FRIES 130

Overview Of The Vegan Diet

Many people who have switched to a vegan diet did so for humanitarian and environmental reasons, in addition to its many health benefits. This is the healthiest way of eating, and numerous studies have shown that vegans have lower chances of developing ailments, including osteoporosis, hypertension, heart difficulties, renal failure, adult-onset diabetes, and arthritis, as well as a decreased risk of becoming obese.

It's also noteworthy that many well-known historical figures turned out to be vegans. Gandhi, Leonardo da Vinci, Charles Darwin, Pythagoras, Benjamin Franklin, and many others are among them.

What are the main arguments for giving up meat and shifting to a plant-based diet? Will you be in the same league as Einstein and da Vinci? Since you have to give up most of your favourite foods and urges, this is not easy.

There will be moments, particularly in the beginning, when you feel like you are at your breaking point. In these dark moments of your vegetarian journey, remember the following rationales for your actions and your need to persevere.

It strengthens the immune system.

It lowers your risk of getting cancers connected to your gender, including breast, prostate, and uterine cancers, as well as cancers of the digestive system.

With meals with little to no fat and adequate energy and satisfaction, a well-balanced vegetarian diet makes you feel full and satisfied. For you to maintain and regulate your weight, this is crucial.

The diet is affordable and will enable you to save money while being tasty and healthy.

You'll be aware that you're contributing to environmental preservation. After all, cattle consume a significant amount of land and water resources. The decrease in animal antibiotic and pesticide residue intake also benefits health.

Many people who identify as vegans have empathy for the suffering that animals endured before being used as food. You can enjoy your food more compassionately when you follow this diet.

Because this type of food doesn't contain cholesterol, it lowers your risk of heart issues.

It takes time and patience to become vegan. Before fully committing to a plant-based diet, you must give your body time to adjust to the changes and see how it reacts.

What to anticipate from this cookbook

This cookbook is intended to give both newbies and older readers all the resources and tools they need to begin increasing the amount of plant-based food in their diets. Here's what to anticipate:

Recipes that are delicious and nutritious: We've made a selection of delectable and nutritious recipes that span breakfast, dinner, snacks, and desserts.

Nutritional data: For you to make well-informed choices about the foods you're putting into your body, we've included nutritional data for each recipe.

Vegan fundamentals: We've provided information on the fundamentals of a vegan diet, such as sources of protein, vitamins, and minerals, and advice on meal planning for individuals new to veganism.

Shopping advice: We've included pointers on how to find vegan-friendly options at the grocery store, such as how to read labels and spot concealed animal components.

Meal planning: To assist you in organising your vegan meals, we've given an example menu with preparation and batch cooking advice.

Useful resources: We've incorporated useful resources throughout the cookbook, like recipe ideas, ingredient replacements, and suggested reading lists for anyone who wants to know more about veganism.

This cookbook is a thorough manual on vegan cooking for novices and older cooks, intended to assist you in learning about the advantages of a plant-based diet and adding more flavorful, nutrient-dense meals to your weekly routine.

Basics Of Veganism

Chapter 1 of this cookbook is dedicated to Vegan Basics, providing a foundation of knowledge for those new to a vegan diet. Here's what you can expect from this chapter:

What is a vegan diet? This section will define a vegan diet and how it differs from other plant-based diets.

Nutrients to focus on: This section will provide an overview of key nutrients to focus on, such as calcium and vitamin B12.

Sources of vegan protein: This section will highlight some of the best plant-based protein sources, including legumes, nuts, and seeds.

Other sources of key nutrients: This section will provide information on other sources of key nutrients, such as iron-rich leafy greens and calcium-rich fortified plant milk.

Vegan substitutes: This section will introduce common vegan substitutes for animal products, such as tofu and tempeh for meat and nutritional yeast for cheese.

Overall, Chapter 1 will provide a thorough understanding of the basics of a vegan diet, laying the groundwork for successful and fulfilling vegan meal planning and preparation.

Comprehending veganism

Adopting a vegan diet and lifestyle requires an understanding of veganism. A philosophy and way of life known as veganism aims to forbid using animals for anything, including clothes, entertainment, food, or any other reason.

The fundamental motivations behind veganism include:

Dedication to animal welfare.

Worries about animal agriculture's effects on the environment.

A vegan lifestyle can be chosen for several reasons, such as ethical, environmental, or health-related.

Legumes, nuts, seeds, fruits, and vegetables. This implies that everything derived from animals—meat, dairy, eggs, and honey, for example—is prohibited. Thankfully, there are now many tasty and healthy plant-based substitutes for these animal products due to the increasing popularity of veganism, making the switch to a vegan diet simpler than ever.

In addition to following a vegan diet, a vegan lifestyle may also entail avoiding leather and wool items and personal care and cleaning products that don't involve animal testing.

Adopting a plant-based diet and lifestyle requires an understanding of veganism, which can also foster a stronger sense of connectedness to the earth and its inhabitants.

How To Make The Switch To A Vegan Diet

But approaching it with the correct attitude and strategy can be a fulfilling and robust experience. To aid with a more seamless transition, consider the following advice:

Begin slowly: Gradually switching to a vegan diet can be beneficial. Start by increasing the amount of plant-based foods you eat, then progressively cut back on the animal products you consume.

Become knowledgeable: Find more about the advantages of a plant-based diet and veganism. This will support you throughout the transfer process to keep you informed and motivated.

Try out some new foods: Try out new dishes and plant-based cuisine. This will keep your new diet from becoming monotonous and help you try new tastes and sensations.

Seek assistance: Make connections with those considering a vegan diet or who are already vegan. This might give you a feeling of belonging and keep you inspired.

Pay attention to nutrient-dense foods: Include nutrient-dense plant-based foods such as legumes, nuts, seeds, whole grains, and leafy greens to ensure that your body is receiving all the nutrients it requires.

Plan your meals: Making a meal plan in advance can help you avoid the urge to grab convenience foods derived from animals and ensure that you always have a range of nutrient-dense plant-based options available.

Remind yourself that adopting a vegan diet is a journey, and making errors or blunders is acceptable. Try not to be too hard on yourself. If you inadvertently ingest animal products, don't punish yourself; instead, see it as a chance to improve.

Switching to a vegan diet requires tolerance, persistence, and an openness to new things. You may effectively switch to a plant-based diet and enjoy all the advantages of leading a vegan lifestyle if you have the appropriate attitude and strategy.

essential components for veganism

Plant-based components are abundant and highly nutritious. The following are essential vegan ingredients to incorporate into your meals:

Fibre and protein. Examples of legumes are kidney beans, black beans, and lentils. They are useful in many recipes, such as burgers, salads, stews, and soups.

Nuts and seeds: Packed full of protein, healthy fats, and minerals like zinc and magnesium, nuts and seeds like cashews, hemp seeds, walnuts, and can be consumed on their own, as a crunchy salad topping, or mixed into smoothies or porridge.

Two great protein sources are tofu and tempeh, both manufactured from soybeans. They work well in various recipes, including sandwiches, curries, and stir-fries.

Minerals like iron and magnesium. Examples of these are quinoa, brown rice, and oats. They work well in salads, stir-fries, and breakfast bowls, among other recipes.

Vegetables: A vegan diet is no different from any other healthy diet in that vegetables are necessary. Rich in vitamins, minerals, and fibre are bright vegetables like bell peppers and sweet potatoes and dark leafy greens like kale and spinach.

Fruits: Rich in natural sweetness, fibre, and antioxidants, fruits are an excellent source of nutrition. Oranges, bananas, apples, and berries are common vegan fruits.

Here are a few examples of plant-based milk that are tasty and nourishing substitutes for dairy milk. They can be eaten on their own or added to recipes.

Plant-based meat substitutes: There are a lot of high-protein plant-based meat substitutes available on the market, including seitan, veggie burgers, and plant-based alternatives to chicken and beef.

These components offer a variety of tastes, textures, and nutritional advantages that can inspire inventive and fascinating vegan cooking. A plant-based diet that is both balanced and healthful can effortlessly include a variety of excellent vegan protein sources.

Chapter 2: Introduction: Making the Switch to a Plant-Based Diet

Chapter 2 transforms into a helpful manual for readers as they embark on their plant-based journey, offering priceless advice and tips to make the switch to a plant-based diet easy. With advice on creating a plant-powered sanctuary in your kitchen and recommendations for a gradual shift, this chapter aims to empower people at every level of their dietary evolution.

Tips for a Gradual Transition

Since switching to a plant-based diet can be a big change for many people, this section focuses on the advantages of taking it step by step. It recognizes that every person's path toward a plant-based diet differs and offers helpful advice for a smooth transition into this revolutionary eating style. Readers are advised to choose a pace that fits their comfort level, whether Meatless Mondays or progressively switching out animal products with plant-based alternatives. Additionally, this section discusses typical transitional problems and provides remedies to help make the process easier to handle.

Provisioning a Plant-Based Kitchen

Ensuring the kitchen is set up to accommodate this dietary change is essential to a smooth transition to a plant-based lifestyle. This section walks readers through the process of assembling a wide variety of plant-based pantry basics. Readers obtain insights into the key components that support plant-based cuisine, from complete grains and legumes to various fruits and veggies.

This section is filled with helpful grocery shopping and meal planning advice to help readers feel confident as they make their way through the aisles. Building a pantry full of herbs, spices, and condiments is a great way to improve the flavour profile of plant-based meals and make the switch healthier and a gourmet adventure.

The Breakfast Sandwich

INGREDIENTS
- 1 cupofgreens (spinach, springmix, greenlettuce, romaine etc.)
- 1-2 medium tomatoes, slicedthin

- 6 pickleslices
- Fresh cracked pepper, totaste
- 1 tablespoonofcoconutoil (orpreferredcookingoil)
- 1 14 ounces of containerextrafirmtofu, pressed& cut lengthwise
- into 6 even slices
- 1 teaspoonofturmeric
- 1/2 teaspoonofgarlic powder
- 1/2 teaspoon of KalaNamak (blacksalt) (subregular salt)
- 3 meltyvegan cheese slices
- 6 slices of bread, 3 orwraps (gluten-free ifpreferred)
- 1-2 tablespoonsofveganmayo

PREPARATION

1. Season tofu on one side with the garlic powder, salt, cracked pepper, and turmeric. Break it out of the ice chamber.
2. Season on the second side
3. When it's time to flip them, put them in the.
4. Skinned on one side, on the pan in a medium pan.
5. Season the upper side while the lower side is cooking.
6. Allow the tofu to cook (for 3 to 5 minutes) until it becomes somewhat crispy and golden.
7. Flip the curtains over and fry the other side for three to five minutes.
8. If preferred, you can pop a cracker in a toaster.

9. Place two pieces of tofu, with a slice of cheese on top of each, on a baking sheet to melt the cheese.

10. Place it in the oven for one to three minutes or until the cheese is melted.

11. You can also use an oven tester.
12. Spread the mustard on both sides of the bread. Place both tofu slices with the cheese on one side and top with the tomatoes.
13. Add a few pinchable lines now and tie the braid together. Reduce the daily amount.

Squishy Chocolate Chipcakes

Ingredients:

- 1 cup coconut sugar
- 1/4 cup maple syrup
- 2 flax eggs (2 tbsp ground flaxseed + 6 tbsp water)
- 1 tsp vanilla extract
- 1 1/2 cups vegan chocolate chips
- 2 cups gluten-free all-purpose flour
- 1 tsp baking soda
- 1/2 tsp salt
- 1 cup coconut oil, melted

Preparation:

1. Place parchment paper on baking sheets.

2. Mixed in a separate, sizable basin.
3. Vegan chocolate chips and stir.

4. After transferring the dough onto the baking pans.
5. Bake it for ten to twelve minutes or until the edges turn golden brown.
6. After a few minutes, let the cookies cool.

Vegan Diet Proven Benefits

Being vegan is not something that appeared out of nowhere one day. It has been around the world in one form or another. The majority of us who live in the modern world find it repulsive to see an animal killed or a living thing in pain.

For most of us, this kind of instinct comes instinctively. We are naturally drawn to a vegan diet because of its many health benefits for our bodies in addition to our disgust of violence.

decreased chance of heart problems

The prevalence of cardiovascular illnesses has sharply grown. Diet, but some can also be placed on our sedentary lifestyle. The typical American diet is heavy in trans fats, cholesterol, saturated fats, and salt. These are all contributing causes of heart disease.

You can easily eliminate cholesterol, trans fats, and saturated fats—three of these four factors—by switching to a vegan diet. The allure of salt is still there, but if you have enough self-control, you can even get rid of it.

lower chance of developing cancer

Our culture is plagued by a lethal toxin called cancer. To be honest, there are a variety of factors for cancer, but nutrition plays a crucial role that cannot be overlooked. It has been demonstrated that low-fat, high-fibre diets, like the vegan diet, lower the risk of malignancies like breast, colon, and prostate cancers.

lower incidence of type 2 diabetes

The diabetes epidemic comes in second to heart disease. Type II diabetes is an acquired illness, whereas type I diabetes is hereditary, sometimes even affecting young children. Simple sugars and carbs in a poor diet can cause blood sugar rises, which increases the risk of insulin tolerance and type II diabetes.

The vegan diet emphasizes the value of natural, unprocessed sources of carbohydrates despite being largely carbohydrate-based. Because the carbohydrates in natural sources are complex, they digest more slowly. They don't result in any sudden increases in blood sugar.

relief from eczema

Many people do not even realize they have a dairy allergy. This allergy is not serious enough to put your life in danger. Most eczema patients and their physicians cannot identify the underlying cause of this skin ailment. They just accept it as things are meant to be and suffer in silence. Removing dairy from their diet can often provide them with unparalleled comfort.

decreased incidence of acne flare-ups

Some individuals may experience moderate allergies like eczema, while others may experience persistent breakouts of acne. Even after you pass the dreaded teenage pimply years behind and into your 20s and 30s. This outbreak may perhaps be a covert allergy of some kind. The most typical allergy is to dairy.

Getting rid of it completely can help you attain the ideal complexion.

more pure breast milk

I mentioned in earlier chapters that livestock animals are raised by injecting hormones into their systems. These changes are transferred to humans when we eat such animals. Such a diet is then transferred to their offspring through the milk of nursing mothers.

Every parent wants to give their kids the best things in life, and what could be better than raw breast milk?

Loss of weight

This is arguably the most well-known advantage, and you have probably heard of it before. The vegan diet can significantly aid in weight loss and waist reduction because it is natural. Due to their high fibre content, fruits, vegetables, and grains help you feel fuller for longer. You won't need to nibble on unhealthy salty and sugary foods as much when you are full. Calorie restriction is essential for the best possible weight loss, but it is simpler to do with a plant-based diet since you feel full and content for longer.

Studies have indicated that shortages in the body may also be the cause of cravings. Your inexplicable cravings will lessen as a vegan diet naturally contains minerals and vitamins. You will undoubtedly grow in better shape over time, even if it takes one step at a time.

Crucial Information On Nutrition

Important nutritional information for a vegan diet; nonetheless, our platform is not equipped to create a comprehensive cookbook for a particular medical condition, like cirrhosis. I can, however, provide some advice regarding the key components that must be present in a cookbook for a vegan cirrhosis diet.

Chronic injury causes the liver to eventually degrade and malfunction, a disease known as cirrhosis. In cirrhosis, it is important to prioritize nutrient-dense foods that support liver health and avoid further damage, even though a vegan diet may benefit general health. A vegan cookbook for the cirrhosis diet should consider a few important factors.

1. Protein Sources: To guarantee a sufficient protein intake, include high-quality plant-based protein sources such as legumes, tofu, tempeh, quinoa, and seitan. Protein is necessary for tissue upkeep and repair, and consuming it in a

carefully balanced diet can help control cirrhosis-related side effects.

2. Complex Carbohydrates: To provide long-lasting energy and vital nutrients like fibre, vitamins, and minerals. These can promote general digestive health and help keep blood sugar levels steady.

3. Healthy Fats: To supply vital fatty acids. These fats also support heart health by lowering inflammation.

4. Vitamins and Minerals: Emphasize foods high in vitamins and minerals, especially those like vitamin E, C, and B-complex vitamins that promote liver function. For a varied nutrient profile, include a range of fruits, vegetables, and leafy greens.

5. Hydration: Stress the value of staying hydrated and provide recipes for drinks high in water, herbs, and fresh fruit juices. Maintaining adequate hydration can promote healthy liver function and aid in removing toxins.

6. Decreased Sodium Consumption: To improve the flavour of food, use less salt and more herbs, spices, and citrus liquids. Reducing sodium consumption can assist in the control of fluid retention and lower the chance of cirrhosis-related complications.

7. Meal Planning and Portion Control: To assist people in maintaining a balanced diet and controlling their calorie consumption, provide advice on meal planning and portion control. Ensure the recipes are adapted to suit the particular dietary demands of people with cirrhosis, considering their particular dietary limitations and preferences.

It's important to keep in mind that people with cirrhosis may have differing degrees of liver damage and require particular diets, so speaking, individualized.

Essential Elements for Handling Cirrhosis

Chronic and progressive liver disease cirrhosis is frequently linked to several risk factors, such as viral hepatitis, non-alcoholic fatty liver disease (NAFLD), and prolonged alcohol use. Cirrhosis can have a major effect on how quickly the illness progresses. Although there isn't a single diet that may treat cirrhosis, concentrating on certain nutrients helps improve liver function, preserve general health, and manage symptoms.

1. Protein: Patients with cirrhosis must consume enough aid in the body's healing process. However, in cirrhosis, the liver's capacity to digest protein may be impaired, resulting in the buildup of harmful byproducts. As a result, it's critical to find a balance and speak with a medical professional to figure out how much protein is right for a person with cirrhosis.

2. Carbohydrates: Blood sugar levels frequently fluctuate in cirrhosis patients. Blood sugar levels and offer a consistent supply of energy. Reducing the consumption of refined carbs and

simple sugars is advised to preserve general health and stop more liver damage.

3. Fat: Keeping your body's fat levels in check is crucial for treating cirrhosis. Consuming a lot of unsaturated fats, such as those in almonds, avocados, and olive oil, can be good for you. These fats can improve general heart health by lowering inflammation. It is essential since they increase the risk of cardiovascular problems and liver damage.

4. Vitamins and Minerals: Patients with cirrhosis frequently exhibit deficiencies in vitamins and minerals due to inadequate nutrient absorption and dietary restrictions. Supplementing with minerals like magnesium and zinc and vitamins like K, D, and E, cirrhosis-related problems.

5. Sodium: Controlling sodium consumption is important for people with cirrhosis since too much salt can cause fluid retention and exacerbate existing problems like oedema and

ascites. Limiting table salt, canned products, and processed foods can help lower sodium intake and relieve associated discomfort.

6. Fluid Intake: People with cirrhosis must be properly hydrated because dehydration can worsen consequences like hepatic encephalopathy. Modify it by each person's unique demands and conditions.

People with cirrhosis should collaborate closely with a physician and a trained dietitian to create a customized nutrition plan that meets their dietary requirements and health objectives. Routine monitoring of liver function and nutritional status is crucial to guarantee the best possible treatment of cirrhosis and stop additional problems.

A Guide to Weight Watchers Pantry Purchases

Let's add a Weight Watchers twist to your grocery shopping to make it easier.

1. Complete Grains:

Eat a lot of whole grains, such as whole wheat pasta, quinoa, and brown rice. Because of their high fibre content, they help you stay full and support your weight management efforts.

2. Trim Proteins:

Pick lean proteins such as beans, fish, tofu, skinless chicken, or turkey. Not only are they pleasant, but they are also brimming with nutrients that your body requires.

3. Fresh Vegetables and Fruits:

Stuff a variety of fruits and vegetables into your trolley. They're loaded with nutrients, low in SmartPoints, and ideal for guilt-free snacking.

4. Low-Satin Milk:

Select dairy products like fat-free or low-fat yoghurt, cheese, and milk. They offer the right amount of creamy richness without packing on the points.

5. Good Fats:

Seize sources of good fats such as olive oil, almonds, and avocados. They keep you feeling full and give your food more flavour.

6. Clever Snacking

Select healthy snacks such as air-popped popcorn, hummus, or Greek yoghurt. They're tasty, filling, and won't stop you in your tracks.

7. Spices and Herbs:

Invest in herbs and spices to enhance flavour without adding additional calories. They're your go-to tactic for adding flavour to nutritious meals.

8. Products in Cans:

Choose canned foods such as tuna, tomatoes, and beans in water. They're adaptable, practical, and ideal for fast, wholesome dinners.

9. Astute Condiments

Seek for flavorful condiments such as balsamic vinegar, spicy sauce, and mustard. They give your foods a little more zest without adding too many points.

10. Heroes of Hydration:

Remember to drink plenty of water! Your hydration heroes are sparkling water, water, and herbal teas.

11. Ice Cream Treats:

Look through the freezer section for quick and wholesome choices. Keep your freezer stocked with lean proteins and fruits. They work well for easy meal prep, stir-fries, and smoothies.

12. Whole Grain Munchies:

Choose full-grain snacks such as crackers made from whole wheat or brown rice cakes. They are filling, crispy, and won't cause you to lose SmartPoints.

13. Protein-Rich Pantry Essentials:

Stock your cupboard with basics high in protein, such as canned beans, lentils, and chickpeas. These are adaptable components that give a dish's protein content a boost.

14. Astute Candies:

Make wise decisions to sate your sweet tooth. Choose dark chocolate, sugar-free gelatin, or fresh fruit. These indulgences will satisfy your appetites without impeding your progress.

15. Eggs:

A flexible and high-protein choice is eggs. They make a simple and quick addition to salads and snacks, or they can be the highlight of a meal.

16. Low-sodium broths:

Use low-sodium broths in your recipes to improve them. They give soups, stews, and sauces depth without using too much salt.

17. Smoked and Grilled Selections:

For proteins like chicken or turkey, consider grilling or smoking them. They enhance the flavour of your food without adding extra calories.

18. Plant-Based Substitutes:

Think about tofu or plant-based burgers as plant-based substitutes. They add diversity and protein to your meals.

19. Rich in Nutrients Cereals:

Select cereals that are low in added sugar and high in nutrients. Combine them with your preferred milk to create a filling breakfast.

20. Conscience Indulgences:

Give yourself a few conscious indulgences. When you want a little something extra, look for sweets that are portion-controlled or have reduced SmartPoint values.

This buying guide lets you stock your pantry with delicious and healthful options. Recall that it's more important to embrace a range of healthful choices supporting your Weight Watchers objectives than to focus only on what you exclude. Happy and astute buying!

You're prepared for success on your Weight Watchers plan with our shopping guide. If you keep it close at hand, you'll be making tasty and informed decisions each time you visit the grocery shop. Cheers to your shopping!

Chapter 3: Take It Easy or Get Rid of It?

I detest discussing calorie counting, so I won't. Still, I will add that if you fully commit to being a vegan (especially a raw vegan), you may not be consuming enough calories each day to meet your body's energy requirements. It won't do to eat two salads and a banana a day! Raw veggies with water content are significantly lower in calories than you might think. You may need more calories even though you consume a lot of them, and for a period, you may feel like you are "eating all the time."

Harmony in Everything

Plan to eat half of your calories from raw plant food, even if you go cooked (nuts are not included). Aim to get half of your daily energy from fruit. For vegans, half of their vegetables should be green, ideally leafy, but use whatever vegetables you find. This implies that most individuals will in a single day than they used to in a week! You will regain your equilibrium, so don't worry.

You may eat Avocados, olives, almonds, and seeds like chia or flax, the highest-fat (and highest-calorie) fruits and veggies. Nevertheless, avoid overindulging in these items on any one day. Alternatively, cut out all of these items the next day if you can overindulge in any of them on a given day. Harmony in everything.

Drinks

Smoothies are a terrific method to gain adequate calories and balance in your vegan diet regularly. Smoothies will not be included in the recipe sections. This is because practically everyone has heard of smoothies, even though most people only associate them with fruit. Smoothies are a great way for vegans, especially those who eat raw food, to consume a lot of vegetables. You can make a smoothie out of any vegetable that you can eat uncooked. Compared to sitting at a large salad bowl and eating the same quantity of whole, raw veggies or fruit, this provides the benefit of packing more vegetables into your body.

The first vegetable smoothie rule is to not expect it to be very sweet! You can anticipate it tasting like vegetables. The second rule for any smoothie, not just vegetable smoothies, is to chew every bite before swallowing. This facilitates the entire digestive system's operation to produce amazing nutrients.

Variety is another element of balance while going vegan. When you were a child, it's possible that your parents only bought carrots, tomatoes, and perhaps iceberg lettuce. You can still experiment now even if you were not exposed to a wide variety of fruits and veggies on your table growing up. To truly understand this kind of variety, imagine your plate to always have some of the following fruits and vegetables:

fresh fruit

greens with leaves

Every meal, serve your greens with four or more other colours and varieties of veggies (except white ones).

sprouts made from pulses or seeds

Sea veggies

Despite what I've just discussed regarding diversity and balance, here's one more piece of advice for making the transition to veganism go smoothly:

In every situation, begin with selecting things you enjoy eating!

For example, if you have never eaten seaweed and don't want to go on this journey, don't do it! Pick something more delicious to eat.

Sleek Out or Gently In?

There are just two approaches to being vegan:

Now is the time to dive straight into this "vegan pool." Everything that isn't a fruit, vegetable, seed, or nut found in Mother Nature should be thrown out or given away. Then, just enjoy cooking delicious meals every day.

Understanding how much food you need to eat each day and what's in your grocery cart, refrigerator, and counters is necessary for the first tactic. You will need to plan out how much of your food will be raw and how much will be cooked, as well as how you will find the time to do so. Planning is essential to ensure that you always have an ample supply of food, particularly when you have to travel for work or become peckish when shopping.

Step gently down from the shallow end of the "vegan pool" and wade cautiously into the deep end. You will still remove all packaged, processed, and refined goods from your fridge, freezer, and cabinets on the No-Go list.

With the second approach, you can pick up where you left off with your eating habits. Are you a meat eater? Do you consume it daily? One way to implement this method would be to consume meat on and off one day. You'll make a cooked vegan dish on the days you don't consume meat. Wean yourself off dairy items similarly if you consume many of them (milk products, cheeses, creams, and yoghurt). Dairy-free on Mondays, minimal on Tuesdays, and so on.

This is an additional iteration of the second tactic. If you want to completely cut out dairy and animal products from your diet, permit yourself to consume meat one day a week and dairy with your meal on another. If your ultimate goal is to live a raw vegan life, set aside another day to cook vegan food. When you perform any of them, your body may just exhale in relief. This strategy might be more effective if you are still consuming any of these banned foods but not in large amounts.

Salad With Couscous

Ingredients

- 1 red bell pepper, chopped
- ½ cup crumbled light feta cheese
- 2⅔ cups water
- 2 tablespoons olive oil
- 2 cups couscous
- ½ cup cucumber, chopped
- 10 cherry tomatoes, sliced in halves
- 2 tablespoons red onion, finely chopped
- ¾ cup dried cranberries

Directions

1. Sauté the couscous for at least five minutes after adding it.
2. Periodically stir, and then pour in the water.
3. Lower the heat and cover the saucepan after the water reaches a boil. Simmer for ten to fifteen minutes.
4. When the couscous is cooked, take it out of the saucepan and transfer it to a bowl

5. Cranberries, red onion, cherry tomatoes, cucumber, and bell pepper should be added.
6. Over the ingredients, drizzle with the herb vinaigrette and toss to combine.
7. Add more feta cheese on top, then serve cold.

Pancakes With Blueberries

Preparation time: 10 minutes

Cooking time: 15 minutes

Number of servings: 4

Ingredients:

- 1/4 teaspoon salt
- 1 cup buttermilk
- 1 large egg
- 2 tablespoons melted butter
- 1 cup fresh or frozen blueberries
- Butter or oil for cooking
- 1 cup all-purpose flour
- 2 tablespoons sugar
- 1 teaspoon baking powder
- 1/2 teaspoon baking soda

Directions:

1. Beat the egg, melted butter, and buttermilk thoroughly in a separate basin.

2. Mix until just mixed, then pour the wet components into the dry ingredients.
3. Avoid overmixing; some lumps are OK.
4. Fold in the blueberries gently.
5. Grease a skillet or griddle with a small amount of butter or oil and heat it.
6. Cook until surface bubbles appear, then turn and cook until golden brown on the other side.
7. Proceed with the leftover batter.
8. Warm pancakes should be served with your preferred toppings or maple syrup.

Why Home-Cooked Food Is More Affordable and Healthier

Many people who begin living a vegan lifestyle discover that cooking most of their meals at home is considerably simpler. There are numerous reasons why cooking at home is more cost-effective and healthier than seeing this as a hardship.

The frugal consumer discovers that cooking at home can result in significant cost savings. Author Laura Stec shows that packing lunches for work is a simple way to save over $100. Cooking at home is even more beneficial because food can be purchased in large quantities, prepared in various ways, and used to save money by store coupons. To make things even simpler, a lot of vegan dishes are excellent for freezing.

The entire amount of time it takes to eat at a restaurant is something that many people overlook. First and foremost, you must make time to gather your family. Arguments over restaurants frequently ensue, with the victorious eatery visible across town through heavy traffic. Then, wait for the server to take your order—even if you live alone. The longest wait begins while you wait for your dinner to be prepared. Then, if you're like most people, you eat quickly because you have somewhere else to be.

At last, you need to take a car home. Cooking at home makes it simple to get rid of all those inconveniences. Even easier is the ability to plan and cook ahead of time if you know you will be busy on a given night.

In many establishments, it is difficult to find vegan options. There are no assurances, even if you take the time to properly examine the menu and consult with the server. Furthermore, food cooked in restaurants typically contains more salt and trans fats. Cooking at home allows you to easily monitor what is in your food, how much fat and salt you consume, and how to prepare it to suit your tastes.

It is necessary to maintain good health. Making balanced meals is considerably simpler when you prepare them at home. In this manner, you may ensure that your diet has the proper protein, vitamin D, vitamin B12, and other vital nutrients.

Every year, food poisoning affects more than 76 million Americans. Making food at home makes it simple to ensure everything is pristine before you start cooking. Additionally, ensuring food is prepared to the correct temperatures and stored correctly is simple.

Eating healthfully gives you enough energy to get through even the most demanding day. Ultimately, it appears that individuals are constantly on the go, from when their alarm clock sounds to well past the recommended bedtime. Adding extra fruit to food prepared at home as a natural pick-me-up is simple, but it is nearly impossible to do so when dining out because the options are typically quite pricey and scarce.

University of Michigan research indicates that eating at home is critical for young individuals. Research indicates that families who share meals regularly have better academic achievement and fewer delinquent issues. Since we are what we eat, cooking at home gives parents the ability to shape their children's future. It is also quite simple for people to include everyone in the cooking process, allowing parents to teach their children valuable lessons about the foods they eat and how to prepare them. Since very few individuals choose to eat vegan food, teaching kids these cooking skills and habits is critical before letting them venture out on their own.

More portions than ever are being served in the majority of eateries. In fact, between 1990 and

2010, the average size of a dinner plate used in a restaurant increased by two inches. When dining out, this encourages consumers to eat more food than they have in the past. At the same time, it is easier for people to manage their portion amounts when they eat at home. As a result, people eat far less food, making it easier for them to manage their weight.

For numerous reasons, preparing meals at home is more cost-effective and healthier than visiting restaurants. When you eat at home, it is incredibly simple to maintain control over what you are putting into your body. You have complete control over the kinds and quantity of food you eat, ensuring that no one goes without what they require. Since you truly are what you eat, you should be in charge of this area of your life rather than a restaurant's chef.

How To Eat A Balanced Diet Without Tracking Calories

I have fantastic news!

You may look and feel fantastic without using a calculator before every meal.

Acquiring the proper nutrition doesn't have to hurt, even though it does involve some planning. I suggest adopting a more laid-back mindset. If you put too much effort into meal planning or monitoring, you will find it difficult to stick to your commitment.

Because the amount of energy that food can provide is expressed in calories, maintaining weight loss requires your body to burn more calories than it receives. Your body won't be driven to burn fat if you eat too many calories and give it more energy than it needs.

To grow muscle, your body requires a lot of protein and an excess of energy to restore and repair itself. Therefore, you need to eat a little more than your body needs to gain weight.

In this chapter, I will provide simple tips to help you consume a healthy diet. By following these guidelines, you'll feel strong and healthy and can gain or lose weight anytime.

ADVERTISE YOURSELF TO EAT ENOUGH

contained in food, and your body uses a lot of energy daily. Energy is necessary for your body to perform many tasks, such as heart beating and food digestion. It must thus be obtained from the meals you eat.

It is, therefore, imperative that you feed your body enough, and this is especially true. Don't be alarmed if you underfeed your body during exercise and find that you don't have the energy to work out hard or feel exhausted overall.

Those working out three or more times a week might use the following math to ensure their body is getting enough time to heal itself.

For every pound of body weight, consume one gram of protein daily. Consume 1.5 grams of carbs daily for every pound of body weight.

One gram of healthy fat or four pounds of excellent fats should be consumed daily.

That's where you should start. It could appear like this for a 130-pound woman: 130 grams of protein daily.

A daily total of 325 grams of fat and 195 grams of carbs.

This equates to about 1,600 calories a day, which should be plenty to progressively increase strength and muscle without gaining weight (which is the goal of "maintenance"—not staying the same).

Vegetarians can easily achieve the objectives above since they can consume a wide range of plant-based proteins and lean protein sources like egg whites and low-fat dairy products. But it gets harder for vegans because the highest protein sources they eat also contain a lot of fats and carbohydrates.

I recommend that vegans eat soy products like tempeh, light and extra-lite tofu, grains (quinoa and amaranth are perhaps the most popular), and legumes (various beans are the most prevalent option here). Vegan protein powders are another helpful supplement, typically blends of proteins from rice, hemp, peas, and other sources.

You will require roughly 20% extra "maintenance" calories. The easiest way to do this is to increase your diet of fats and carbs (fats have nine calories per gram, whereas carbohydrates only have 4).

You should reduce your "maintenance" calories by about 20% to lose weight. The easiest way to achieve this is to reduce carbohydrate intake. You should put a lot of effort into eating well-balanced meals. Junk food that lacks nutrients, such as white bread, chips, soda, and juice, may make you lose weight temporarily, but it is not a healthy way to lose weight and will eventually catch up with you.

Conversely, calorie-dense foods like fruits, vegetables, healthy grains, and premium meats will keep your body in top physical shape.

EAT ENOUGH QUALITY PROTEIN.

You need more protein in your diet than the average person. Why? Because muscular damage from exercise is repaired with protein.

The "micro-tears" that each repetition causes in your muscle fibres are repaired by your body. But in addition to returning them to their original state, the body grows them bigger and stronger so they can endure the stress of exercise.

You need to eat enough high-quality protein to reap the full benefits of your exercise regimen. And it extends beyond simply overindulging in meals following a workout. It means reaching your daily objective, regardless of whether you do it in three or seven meals.

These days, the two main protein sources are whole food protein and supplement protein.

As you may have guessed, whole-food protein comes from organic foods like eggs, cottage cheese, and quinoa. For whole-food protein, your best bets should be quinoa, low-fat Greek yoghurt, tempeh, tofu, eggs, almonds, rice, and beans.

Some people argue that you must carefully combine your proteins if you're a vegetarian or vegan to ensure that your body gets "complete" proteins, including all of the amino acids needed to make tissue. Although this idea is still commonly believed, the American Dietetic Association has disproved it as a myth and the defective study it was based on. There is evidence that some vegetable protein sources are not as rich in particular amino acids as other protein sources, but this does not mean they are entirely lacking.

The three most widely used protein supplement sources are soy, whey (the liquid after milk is curdled and pressed to make cheese), and eggs. Protein supplements are meals that come in powder or liquid form and contain protein from different sources. Furthermore, fantastic plant-based supplements contain high-quality protein sources, including fruit, quinoa, brown rice, peas, and hemp.

To eat healthily, you don't need protein supplements, but since you'll be consuming protein four to six times a day, some people might find it impractical to get all their protein from whole foods.

There are a few things you should know before consuming. It is the first thing to worry about. Because the subject is so complex, studies on it are very ambiguous and contentious. Your metabolism, digestion, genetics, lean mass, and lifestyle all have a big impact. We know you can use it, but let's be clear. Exactly how much? More than 100 grams at once should be easily digested by your body, though.

It's helpful to know this even if there are no benefits to eating this way (I find overloading rather uncomfortable). This way, you can make up for missing a meal by putting on more protein at a later meal.

Moreover, the body absorbs certain proteins more efficiently than others, and different proteins break down at different rates. The body can readily absorb whey protein and utilize up to 90% of what you eat, thanks to its "net protein utilization" (NPU) in the low 90% range. Egg protein has an NPU similar to whey's while digesting much more slowly than whey.

Chapter 4: Filling Bowls & Salads

Salads were an afterthought for many years before switching to a plant-based diet; they were a green side dish that was obediently combined to appear healthy before indulging in the "main event" of an animal-centred meal. How silly I feel now that I know how abundant Salad may be! Since adopting vegan, green dishes have evolved into vibrant, filling meals that prioritize nutrition above superfluous proteins.

My affinity with produce grew as green gems transformed from simple icebergs into internationally inspired medleys highlighting seasonal nutrients. Instead of being used as lone garnishes, kale became a cosy sauté alongside grains and beans. However, constructing harmonious, mouthwatering bowls necessitated abandoning outdated notions of "salad" as an afterthought. My ability to experiment led me to develop meals that, with every satisfying bite, harmonize body, soul, and values.

To start, I would only add canned chickpeas or edamame to baby spinach, along with crunchy cucumbers, radishes, and snow peas. Soon, local and international cuisines influenced concoctions like Israeli couscous mixed with sun-dried tomatoes, kalamata olives, and artichoke hearts, or zesty Thai noodle salad with shredded carrots, chopped peanuts, and a lime-ginger vinaigrette. Without dairy or meat, nutritious toppings like nutritional yeast, hemp seeds, or pumpkin seeds offered protein, creaminess, and richness.

Zesty "noodles" dominated late-summer harvests, tucked under ribbons of basil and squash blossoms tossed in a light vinaigrette. A spicy chipotle aioli complemented the warm bowls of quinoa, black beans, and roasted corn, creating a layered dish of delight. And when the temperature dropped, creamy tahini dressing paired with crispy Brussels sprouts and cabbage topped with steaming heaps of farro for hearty comfort food.

The most satisfying were dishes that brought flavours from overseas with every bite. Seaweed salad, edamame, and shiitake mushrooms are combined with sushi rice to make Japanese rice bowls. Middle Eastern delicacies stacked pita bread, hummus, roasted cauliflower, and tabbouleh for hand-held enjoyment. Simple combo meals, such as crackers with marinated artichoke hearts and arugula pesto that was delicious with every mouthful, still provided diversity. Defying the conventions of salad dressings allowed worldly wonders to be included in cosy dishes that fed the body and the spirit.

Whether it's working parents longing for home-cooked dinners or students yearning for handy campus food, sharing vegan tweaks motivated pals to adopt better lifestyles; together, we found that eating doesn't have to mean sacrificing animal products. The most important factors were accessibility and simplicity, allowing vegetables to be placed alongside superfoods like grains and legumes. I wish the upcoming version of Salad would promote compassionate well-being everywhere!

Here are some of my favourite hearty Salad and bowl recipes that showcase seasonal ingredients, all in the spirit of fostering connection and compassion via plant-centric cooking. I hope they provide you solace and motivation as your connection to produce grows. Playing is fun, so don't be scared to try new things; that's where the delights of nourishment reside. Forward to several auspicious dinners surrounded by the abundance of our planet!

Why Make The Vegan Switch?

Naturally, the main query is: Why should we become vegans and give up meat? Plenty of strong moral, ethical, environmental, and health arguments exist for giving up meat in your diet. But before we get into each of those reasons in more detail, let's take a closer look at the role that meat plays in our society today to better understand why it's so crucial to make the ethical decision to become vegan.

The Custom of Meat

There's no denying that eating meat has become a staple of many of our life's major celebrations. Meat has come to be associated in a certain way with festivities. Consider it. Turkey is frequently the first food that comes to mind when we mention Thanksgiving. Conversely, ham frequently takes centre stage as the customary Easter dinner. Then, when summer arrives, many hungry mouths eagerly await the first steak or burger to be cooked on the grill.

But as a species, humans most likely evolved to consume fruits, vegetables, nuts, berries, and legumes. We are more similar to herbivorous animals than carnivorous ones in terms of how our jaws and teeth are shaped, the muscles in our faces, and the saliva in our mouths.

How did we regard meat as a staple of our festivals if our natural diet was planted?

We can assume that the first intake of flesh was an act of self-preservation motivated by the urge to survive. It was natural that early male groups would resort to meat when they became hunter-gatherers because of the abundance of resources, the flavour of cooked meat, and the long-lasting energy that comes from meat's high fat content. It is possible that under these conditions, meat first became a staple of social gatherings.

For example, in earlier days, discovering cooked meat from a forest fire would have been a source of great joy, and entire clans would have shared in that lucky windfall. Meat played a significant role in the wider scheme of community life back then. For example, hunting was typically a cooperative activity in which groups tracked, pursued, and ultimately killed their target.

The outcome of these hunts meant food for the hunter and the many other clan members who depended on the hunters for survival. Whole clans depended on the success of these hunts. Therefore, the sight of meat would have been met with applause by those who waited for the hunters to return because it meant they could stuff their bellies for another day. It would have also required teamwork to skin the animal and chop or tear the meat from the carcass after it was returned to the tribe. Everyone would have taken part in this and reaped their labour's benefits together. Therefore, it's simple to understand how meat came to be associated with gathering and celebration—a necessity engrained in our societies. With family and friends, we commemorate the numerous seasons and life milestones. Since eating meat was a common part of early human festivities, this custom has persisted into the present era.

The issue is that food ought to fuel and nourish the body while providing energy and renewal. Like any machine, the human body needs the correct fuel to function at its best. Our bodies that suffer from hypertension, type 2 diabetes, or hypercholesterolemia are similar to automobile engines that aren't properly tuned or aren't using the right kind of gasoline. Like automobiles, our bodies require the proper fuel to function at their best. Furthermore, the human body was not designed to function on high-fat or antibiotic-fed meat. Fortunately, you can nourish your body the right way with a vegan diet. Eating veganism is like filling up your automobile with the best, highest-grade gasoline money can buy. Eating unhealthy meat is like putting improper diesel fuel in your sparkling sports car that damages its engine.

Associated with eating meat, let's discuss some of the most convincing arguments in favour of switching to a vegan diet.

Reasons related to health

To put it plainly, eating a good vegan diet is far healthier. Numerous academic research studies and firsthand accounts have demonstrated the remarkable health benefits of a plant-based diet.

Diseases When it comes to diseases, being a vegan can help keep our bodies free of disease. Changing to a plant-based diet can improve your health in many ways. In this section, we'll talk about how veganism can help with many issues associated with some of the most prevalent medical disorders that affect people today.

Heart Conditions

Research indicates that vegans have much lower risks, lower cholesterol, and a decreased likelihood of blood pressure problems. Diets low in saturated fat, which can be converted to cholesterol, are vegan. In consequence, cholesterol clogs arteries and restricts blood flow, which causes heart disease and strokes. Vegan diets completely sidestep this issue because they almost completely lack cholesterol.

Even though fat is necessary for good health, vegans have an advantage since they use unsaturated fat, found in plant oils like coconut and olive oils and primarily derived from seeds. Moreover, soluble fibre, generally present in vegetables, whole grains, and beans, among other foods, is also abundant in vegan diets. Soluble fibre contributes to the health and happiness of vegans by absorbing a large amount of the harmful cholesterol that ultimately damages our bodies.

Finally, plants have compounds that benefit us. Phytosterols and other antioxidants in various fruits and vegetables help prevent heart disease. In summary, going vegan is the best option to maintain a healthy heart for years to come!

Let them cool somewhat before arranging to serve.

Once the baking sheet is ready, place a rounded dough scoop on it. Bake for 10 to 12 minutes or until golden brown. Health And Inflammation

Although they may seem complicated, let's simplify inflammatory disorders. Think of your body as a stronghold that keeps you safe from attackers.

Like your body's warning system, inflammation activates when something isn't right. This is generally beneficial because it aids in recuperating from injuries.

But occasionally, this alarm system gets a little too excited. What if a leaf blew by and set off your house alarm each time? That's comparable to what occurs in certain disorders when there is inflammation. Inflammatory illnesses resemble internal wars within your body where an alarm system continually goes off, harming rather than assisting.

Our bodies' defences may erode with age, leaving us more susceptible to these conflicts. Seniors may, therefore, occasionally be more susceptible to inflammatory illnesses. Such disorders include, among others, diabetes (when blood sugar becomes unstable), heart disease (when blood vessels in the heart become clogged), and arthritis (when your joints pain and swell). For seniors, they may make living more difficult and impact their ability to move, feel, and enjoy life.

➤ Inflammatory Symptoms

1. Pain and Swelling: If your body were a map, the pain would be the "X", designating the location. Inflammation can occasionally result in pain and swelling in bodily areas like muscles or joints. This can make getting about a little challenging.

2. Redness and Warmth: Have you ever unintentionally touched a warm stove? When inflammation occurs, certain areas of your body may feel warmer or appear redder than usual. It seems to be your body's method of alerting you to an issue.

3. Experiencing Fatigue: Envision yourself as a superhero who has spent the entire day engaged in combat. I assume you'd be exhausted. Indeed, inflammation can resemble those conflicts. It may cause fatigue even in the absence of extreme physical exertion.

4. Difficulty Breathing or Digesting: Inflammation can occasionally lead to invisible issues in areas of the body, such as the stomach

or lungs. It could cause you to feel queasy or have trouble breathing.

5. Modifications to Your Appearance and Feeling: Skin inflammation may cause changes to the appearance of your skin. Alternatively, it could interfere with your memory recall. It's as if your body is telling you something isn't quite right.

➤ Reasons for Inflammation

Influencers of Lifestyle and Inflammation

Think of your body as a garden. Just like plants need adequate care to thrive, so does your body. If you don't get enough sleep, aren't physically active, or are always stressed out, you're not giving your garden the right conditions to flourish. Inflammation may result from these substances.

Stress: Imagine that stress is the evil guy trying to wreck everything, and your body is the superhero. Your body releases chemicals when under stress, which may exacerbate inflammation. Stated differently, it's akin to inviting the antagonist into your yard!

Not getting enough sleep Sleep has a profound effect on your body. It allows your body to repair and rejuvenate. Your body's immune system may not work as well when you don't get enough sleep, which could allow inflammation to develop.

Absence of Exercise: Your body is naturally gregarious. Similar to how a car must be driven to maintain its condition. Your body's capacity to combat inflammation may become a little sluggish when you don't exercise enough, which allows inflammation to spread.

Dietary Factors Associated with Prolonged Inflammation

Now let's talk about the meals you eat. Food is fuel for your body, but not all fuels are equal. Certain meals are like friends who help your body stay strong, but other meals might be like enemies that worsen inflammation.

Sugar-filled sweets and processed foods: Consider your body to be a machine. If you feed it too many processed foods and sugars, sand is pouring into the gears. These foods can potentially raise your body's level of inflammation, which can lead to several problems.

Unhealthy fats Although fats are necessary for your health, some fats are better than others. Think of the body as the engine of a car. Good fats maintain an engine operating smoothly, much like premium oil does. Bad fats are like old, dirty oil; they can make inflammation flare up.

Overindulgence in Meat: Meat may be delicious, but consuming too much of it may not be wise. Certain meats, especially red and processed meats, may make inflammation worse. It's similar to adding gasoline to an already flaming inflammatory fire.

Insufficient Vegetables and Fruits: Think of your body as a garden. Vegetables and fruits are comparable to the vivid flowers that enhance the appearance of your yard. Their high vitamin and antioxidant content can help lower inflammation.

Favorably impacts both the environment and their health.

The Foundations Of High-Protein Vegan Dietary Plans

Concerns about animal welfare, sustainability of the environment, and health have all contributed to the notable increase in interest in and adoption of veganism in recent years. But with the traditional connection between protein and animal products, a significant worry for people switching to a vegan diet is how much protein they get. This chapter tries to give readers a thorough grasp of a vegan high-protein diet. It covers important nutrients, foods high in plant-based protein, ways to balance macronutrients, and how to get the recommended amount of protein each day.

Crucial Elements in a Plant-Based Diet

A well-balanced vegan diet should consist of a range of nutrient-dense foods to guarantee that the body gets the necessary nutrients. Crucial elements for vegans consist of:

Protein: Needed for hormone production, enzyme function, and tissue growth and repair. Plant-based protein sources include legumes (beans, lentils, peas), tofu, tempeh, seitan, nuts, seeds, and grains.

DNA synthesis and neuron function. Vegans should consider B12 supplements or fortified meals like plant-based milk and morning cereals, even though B12 is frequently found in animal products.

Iron: Required for the blood's oxygen delivery system. Lentils, beans, tofu, spinach, and fortified cereals are plant-based iron sources, with foods high in iron to improve absorption.

Calcium: Vital for strong bones. Almonds, tofu, fortified plant milk, and leafy green vegetables are vegan sources.

Omega-3 Fatty Acids: Vital to the health of the heart and brain. Algae-based supplements, walnuts, chia seeds, and flaxseeds are vegan sources.

Zinc: Requires both wound healing and immunological activity.

High Protein Plant-Based Diets

Contrary to popular belief, well-planned plant-based diets can be high in protein. Several top-notch sources of plant-based protein consist of:

Legumes: A cheap, adaptable, and high-protein staple, including beans, lentils, and peas.

Tempeh and tofu are soy-based products that can be used in various recipes and are great protein sources.

It is versatile and may be used in many savoury recipes.

Nuts and Seeds: Rich in protein, almonds, peanuts, chia seeds, and hemp seeds these also offer critical nutrients and healthy fats.

Whole Grains: Nutritious grains that boost protein consumption include quinoa, brown rice, bulgur, and oats.

Macronutrient Balancing for Optimal Health

Although a vegan diet must include protein, maintaining a balance between macronutrients—proteins, fats, and carbohydrates—is critical for good health. A balanced vegan diet consists of:

Proteins: A varied amino acid profile is ensured by including a range of meals in addition to plant-based protein sources. To improve the balance of amino acids, eat complementary proteins like grains and beans.

Fats: It is essential for brain function and the absorption of fat-soluble vitamins to include.

Carbohydrates: Legumes, fruits, vegetables, and whole grains offer a consistent supply of vital nutrients and energy.

Little Carrot Cakes For Breakfast

Prep time: 15 minutes
Cooking time: **12 minutes**
Servings: **6**

Ingredients:

- 1 ½ cup of rice milk
- 1 teaspoon baking powder
- 2 tablespoon flax meal
- 1 tablespoon pumpkin seeds
- 1 teaspoon coconut oil
- 1 cup water, for cooking
- 2 carrots, grated
- 1 banana, mashed
- 4 tablespoon brown sugar

- 1 cup all-purpose flour
- 1 teaspoon vanilla extract

Directions:

1. Combine the mashed banana and the grated carrot in the mixing bowl.
2. Add the flax meal, flour, and baking powder after that.
3. Add rice milk and continue to stir until the mixture is smooth.
4. Remix it.
5. After using coconut oil to coat the moulds, fill the mini cake moulds with the carrot mixture.
6. Fill the instant pot with water and place the steamer trivet on top.

7. Line the trivet with the moulds, then cover with foil. Using a toothpick, poke medium-sized holes in the foil and secure the edges.
8. Shut the cover and select the Manual (High pressure) setting.
9. For 12 minutes, cook the cakes. After that, quickly relieve the pressure for ten minutes.
10. After taking off the foil, cool the cakes to room temperature.

Breakfast Burrito For Vegans With Tofu Scramble

Ingredients:

- 1/2 teaspoon chili powder
- Salt and pepper to taste
- 1 can black beans, drained and rinsed
- 4 whole-grain tortillas
- 1 block firm tofu, crumbled
- 1 tablespoon olive oil
- 1 teaspoon cumin
- Salsa, avocado slices, and fresh cilantro for topping

Instructions:

1. Crumbled tofu should be pan-fried in olive oil until it begins to brown.
2. Blend thoroughly.
3. Add the black beans and heat through, stirring.

4. Heat the whole-grain tortillas in the microwave or on a dry skillet.
5. Fill each tortilla with a spoonful of the tofu and black bean mixture.
6. Add slices of avocado, fresh cilantro, and salsa on top.
7. Create a delectable vegan breakfast burrito by folding the tortilla's edges.
8. Enjoy the delicious plant-based meal while it's hot!

Creating A Helpful Network

As a vegan advocate, it is imperative to surround oneself with a supportive network. Here's how to accomplish it:

1. To meet people who share your ideals, join vegan organizations online and in your community. Speaking with others who share your values about your experiences and recommendations could be empowering.

2. Teach Your Close Circle: Talk to your loved ones and close friends about your decision and why it is important. People who understand your viewpoint tend to become your biggest supporters.

3. Ask a Practitioner for plant-based nutrition assistance if you have health or nutritional problems while following a vegan diet. They might offer personalized suggestions to ensure your diet is well-balanced and satisfies your nutritional needs.

Eating a Vegan Diet and Staying Well

Avoiding Dietary Mistakes and Consulting Medical Experts

When followed appropriately, a vegan diet may offer several health benefits. Like any nutritional choice, there are risks associated with it as well.

This section discusses some common nutritional issues and stresses the importance of seeing a healthcare professional to maintain optimal health when on a vegan diet.

Possible Hazards to Nutrition

1. Protein Intake: Obtaining adequate protein may worry some vegans. Tempeh should be consumed to meet protein requirements.

2. Vitamin B12: The majority of vitamin B12 comes from animal sources, therefore vegans require it. Think about using supplements or fortified foods to prevent deficiencies.

3. Iron: Although there are many plant-based sources of iron, their absorption might not be as efficient as that of animal sources. Iron-rich

meals may be better absorbed when combined with vitamin C-rich foods.

4. Leafy greens, fortified meals, and plant-based milk are good sources of calcium. Ensure that your intake meets your needs for the day.

5. Omega-3 Fatty Acids: While walnuts, chia seeds, and flaxseeds are good sources of omega-3s, some people choose to take supplements made of algae to ensure proper absorption.

6. Zinc: Consume foods high in zinc, needs.

7. Iodine: Seaweed and iodized salt may contain iodine, but too much iodine from seaweed may be harmful.

Chapter Two: Nutritional Considerations

For vegans, paying attention to specific nutrients is important to achieve optimal nutrition. Vegans must eat fortified foods or take supplements to obtain vitamin B12, often found in animal sources. Leafy greens and plant-based milk fortified with calcium are good sources. Meals high in vitamin C are superior for absorbing iron derived from plant sources.

The macronutrients—carbs, proteins, and fats—must be balanced. All the elements needed may be found in a well-planned vegan diet, but it's important to consider portion sizes, food diversity, and dietary restrictions.

In summary, abstaining from animal products is part of a vegan diet for moral, ecological, and health reasons. It encourages a plant-based diet and comprises. By carefully planning their diets and attending to specific nutritional variables, vegans can maintain a healthy and well-balanced lifestyle while lessening their influence on the entire planet and its inhabitants.

All animal products—including dairy, eggs, meat, and even honey—are prohibited in a vegan diet. Nuts and seeds make up the majority of it. This meal choice is becoming increasingly well-liked because of its numerous, well-established health benefits.

1. Cardiovascular Health: Heart disease risk has been associated with a vegan diet. Two substances that can clog arteries and lead to atherosclerosis.

The high fibre content of plant-based meals also helps to regulate blood pressure.

2. Weight Control: Vegan diets often promote weight loss and control. Their higher fibre and lower calorie content help control appetite and prevent overindulgence. Moreover, emphasizing whole, unprocessed meals may promote healthy eating practices.

3. Lower Cancer Risk: Research has shown that vegans have a lower risk of developing some cancers, such as prostate, breast, and colon cancer. Phytochemicals and antioxidants can prevent the development of cancer.

4. Better Blood Sugar Control: Vegan diets benefit

Diets based on plants contain complex carbs, which are digested more slowly and lower blood sugar spikes. Additionally, some studies indicate that vegan diets could enhance insulin sensitivity.

5. Digestive Health: The high fibre content of vegan meals promotes digestive health. In addition to encouraging regular bowel movements, fibre may reduce the chance of developing conditions like diverticulitis, constipation, and irritable bowel syndrome.

6. Lower Cholesterol Levels: This promotes general cardiovascular health and reduces the risk of atherosclerosis.

7. Longevity: Several extensive studies have shown that vegans may have longer lifespans than those who eat animal products. This possible benefit is largely attributed to the decreased risk of chronic disorders.

A well-balanced vegan diet requires careful preparation to ensure enough consumption of essential minerals, including vitamin B12, vitamin D, calcium, iron, and omega-3 fatty acids. Speaking with a medical professional or registered dietitian allows people to follow a vegan diet while still meeting their nutritional needs. A vegan diet offers several health advantages.

Section 1: Definition of Veganism

One way to refer to a particular vegetarian diet is "veganism." Meat, eggs, dairy products, and any other substance produced from animals are not allowed in a vegan diet. This includes items like white sugar and some varieties of wine that have been processed with animal products. The only foods that can be consumed on this diet are plant-based items.

A person following these dietary requirements is called a vegan. 'Vegan' also refers to a type of food.

Being vegan can be motivated by several factors, such as ● Wanting to live a generally healthier lifestyle, ● Wanting to avoid animal cruelty and death, ● Wanting to lose weight, ● Reducing the toxic overload climate and environment, ● Fighting world hunger by feeding crops to less fortunate people instead of farm animals.

● Letting animals live in their native environments, free from human interference.

Three different vegan diets exist:

● Plant-based veganism: Most adopters of this vegan diet do so to improve their health or to reduce their body weight. They decide not to eat dairy or meat. Consequently, the diet has cleared all saturated fats, encouraging weight loss and better health. This diet is well-liked since it is simple to follow, contributes to preventing chronic illnesses like type 2 diabetes and heart disease, and has a smaller environmental impact.

- Raw veganism: This vegan diet excludes anything heated or cooked. As a result, the primary foods in this diet are fruits, vegetables, grains, nuts, and seeds. Once more, the main reason this diet was chosen is its health benefits. Some make this decision for spiritual reasons, thinking they are building a new Garden of Life or Eden. There are various approaches to veganism. The first eats 80% of it according to the 80/10/10 rule. Alternatively, you can follow the "raw till 4" vegan diet, which entails eating raw food until 4 p.m. and then having a cooked meal for dinner.
- Veganism that is High Carb Low Fat (HCLF): As the name implies, followers of this kind of veganism will eat as little fat as possible and a lot of carbs in the form of fruits, vegetables, and grains. Additionally, practitioners might choose healthy fats like avocados, seeds, nuts and carbohydrates like potatoes, grains, and pasta. This is the path that many new vegans pursue

since it makes the transition easier and allows them to eat a nutritious, balanced diet without as many constraints as raw or plant-based veganism.

This book will concentrate on information and recipes that align with the plant-based vegan diet.

Vegetarian vs. Vegan

The phrases "vegan" and "vegetarian" are sometimes used synonymously, making it difficult for someone who is just starting as a vegan to distinguish between the two. Even though neither diet allows meat, they are not equivalent.

Although vegetarians abstain from meat, they still eat dairy products like milk and eggs. Vegans, on the other hand, don't use any animal products or leftovers. In other words, vegans do not eat any animal products at all, whereas vegetarians refrain from eating meat but occasionally may use dairy or eggs.

Vegetarianism comes in various forms. Among them are:

- Vegetarianism that is lacto-ovo: This is the most prevalent kind. Lacto-ovo vegetarians consume dairy and eggs but abstain from meat, poultry, and shellfish.
- Lacto vegetarianism: People who follow this diet avoid eggs, meat, poultry, and shellfish but consume dairy products.
- Ovo vegetarianism: People who practice this diet consume eggs but refrain from consuming dairy, meat, poultry, or shellfish.
- Pesco vegetarianism: This kind of vegetarianism deviates from the norms since its adherents still consume fish and other seafood but abstain from meat and fowl.

While vegetarianism is solely a nutritional decision, veganism also refers to various lifestyle choices beyond your food choices, such as the products you use, the materials your home is constructed of, and lifestyle items.

Regardless of the rationale behind adopting a vegan diet, the fundamental aspect is that no animal products are purchased or consumed.

Is Veganism a Diet or a Way of Life?

Most vegans define veganism more broadly than simply following their dietary restrictions. This also includes the items they decide to buy for use and the goods they use in their homes. For this reason, the definition of veganism has been expanded to encompass a lifestyle that, to the greatest extent feasible, abstains from all forms of animal abuse and exploitation. Most people opt to live vegan lifestyles because of this ethical consideration.

The majority of vegans avoid using leather, fur, wool, and cosmetics that either contain animal materials or are subjected to animal testing. They even choose not to visit zoos and aquariums.

Many also decide to adopt a vegan diet to lessen their environmental effect. Numerous environmental consequences result from animal farming, including clearing forests to make room for the practice, removing plant materials from human consumption to feed livestock, transporting animals, releasing greenhouse gases into the atmosphere, and many more. In addition to lowering deforestation and other acts that benefit the environment rather than put undue strain on it, becoming vegan also helps to lessen the carbon footprint that humans leave behind.

Thus, if you're considering becoming vegan, consider it because it involves a lifestyle change and dietary adjustments.

Accepting The Shift: A Guide To Lectin-Free Vegan Transition

Are you prepared to go on a vegan diet devoid of lectins? Welcome to the team! While the path holds bright benefits, the first step can be like navigating a foreign forest. But do not be alarmed, bold adventurer! With the help of this guide, you will be able to navigate the shift and thrive on your plant-powered journey.

1. Fill Up Your Lectin-Lite Cabinet:

Like any intrepid traveller needs a fully equipped bag, your lectin-free pantry needs some TLC, too. To get you started, here are some essentials you must have:

Leafy Greens: Rich in vitamins and fibre, collard greens, kale, and spinach are the leafy companions of your digestive system.

Vibrant Fruits: Citrus fruits, melons, and berries are nature's candies, rich in antioxidants and low in lectins.

Healthy Fats: No drama with lectins—fuel your body and taste buds with avocados, olives, and coconut oil.

Nut and Seed Butter: Sunflower, cashew, and almonds are powerful sources of taste and protein; choose roasted or soaked types to minimize lectins.

Lectin-Friendly Legumes: Black beans, green beans, and lentils are lower in lectins than their brethren while offering important protein and fibre.

Whole Grains: Quinoa, brown rice, and millet are complex carbohydrates that provide long-term energy without gluten-related lectins.

Herbs & spices: flavour without the hassle; liven up your meals with diversity and excitement.

2. Learn to Use the Meal Plan Manoeuvre:

A plan is the first step towards conquering mealtime mayhem. Here are some tips for making tasty meals that consider lectins:

Weekly Meal Planning: Set aside some time weekly to plan your meals, making grocery shopping much easier.

Love Leftovers: Tap into the Power of Remaining Food! Save time and energy by cooking double batches and enjoying them for lunch or another meal.

Snack Savvy: When feeling peckish, keep lectin-friendly snacks like almonds, apples, or vegetable sticks on hand.

Batch Cooking Bliss: To make quick and delicious meals, simply prepare grains, legumes, and roasted veggies ahead of time.

Be Creative: Try new dishes, play with tastes, and enjoy yourself in the kitchen!

3. Conquering the Tigers of Transition:

Adopting a new diet frequently raises questions and presents difficulties. Here's how to overcome a few typical obstacles on your path away from lectin:

Nutrient Deficiencies: Discuss potential dietary requirements and supplements, if necessary, with your physician or a certified dietitian.

Social Situations: Bring lectin-free food to potlucks and restaurant gatherings, or gently explain your dietary restrictions while mingling with others.

Requirements and Persuasion: Avoid starving yourself! Arrange special occasions and concentrate on the long-term advantages and delectable substitutes.

Changes in Digestion: Give your stomach some time to adapt! Minimizing initial discomfort can be achieved by gradually transitioning and maintaining hydration.

4. Discovering the Lectin-Free Group:

It's more enjoyable to travel with pals! Here are several places you may go to meet and hear from other vegans who avoid lectins:

Interests: sign up for forums, Facebook groups, or online courses.

Blogs and Websites: Look through lectin-free vegan blogs' and websites' recipes, advice, and inspiration.

Books & Cookbooks: For in-depth information and mouthwatering recipes, peruse the works of chefs or nutritionists who specialize in the lectin-free vegan diet.

Support Groups: To exchange experiences and gain knowledge from others, contact your neighbourhood support groups or attend seminars.

Remember that changing your diet is a marathon, not a sprint. Above all, remember to enjoy the trip and practice self-compassion. Reward yourself for little accomplishments. You'll be smiling and confidently navigating the lectin-free vegan jungle in no time, enjoying the benefits of a happy and healthy existence with a dash of drive and these pointers. Let's explore the world of delicious recipes and turn your plate into a feast of delicious gut-healing foods!

LABEL READING AND DETERMINING HIDDEN INGREDIENTS

1. Recognize Terminology Used in Labeling:

Making educated decisions starts with reading labels.

Learn the terms used on labels for vegan and gluten-free products. Seek certifications like

"Gluten-Free" or "Certified Vegan" to ensure the product satisfies your dietary needs.

2. Check for Information on Allergens:

Explore the facts about allergens. Gluten can be found under many names, such as wheat, barley, or rye. In a similar vein, non-vegan components could show up as unidentified animal byproducts. Terms like "whey" and "casein" or "gelatin" should be avoided.

3. Verify for Inherent Contamination:

Cross-contamination can happen during processing, even if a product is labelled as vegan or gluten-free. Look for labels like "Processed in a facility that handles dairy" or "May contain traces of gluten."

Choose items with specific gluten-free and vegan facilities if you suffer from severe allergies.

4. Watch Out for Hidden Sugars:

Vegan or gluten-free snacks may contain sugar to make up for their flavour. Look past the word "sugar" on the label and take caution when reading names like malt syrup, agave nectar, or high-fructose corn syrup.

For a healthy option, choose snacks that are low in added sugar or have natural sweeteners.

5. Assess Synthetic Additives:

Certain vegan and gluten-free snacks could have artificial taste enhancers in them.

Look for additives such as flavourings, colours, or artificial preservatives. Selecting snacks with few, easily recognized ingredients guarantees a healthier and more hygienic choice.

Natural remedies for Crohn's disease

people to help, including Crohn's disease.

These are for use in treatment; however, some individuals use them in addition to prescription drugs.

Avoid adding new treatments to your current regimen without first seeing your physician.

Among the CAM treatments for Crohn's disease include:

Probiotics. These are live bacteria that can assist you in replenishing and reestablishing healthy bacteria in your digestive tract. Additionally, probiotics may aid in preventing bacteria from upsetting your gut's natural balance and resulting in a Crohn's disease flare-up. Specific information regarding limited effectiveness.

Probities. These are potentially helpful materials in plants like asparagus, bananas, carrots, and leeks. They help nourish and multiply the friendly bacteria in your stomach.

Fish oil. Fish oil can be found in omega-3. According to a 2017 study, research on the potential treatments for Crohn's disease, such as mackerel and salmon, is still ongoing. Fish oil supplements are available online.

Supports. Many people think certain herbs, vitamins, and minerals can alleviate symptoms of many illnesses, including inflammation associated with Crohn's disease. Research on which supplements might be beneficial is still ongoing.

Aloevera. Some people believe that the aloe vera plant possesses anti-inflammatory effects. As one of the main causes of Crohn's disease, inflammation can be used as a natural anti-inflammatory. But currently, no research suggests that Crohn's disease can also be treated with vera.

Chinese medicine. This is the technique of carefully inserting needles into the skin to trigger various body points. According to a 2014 study, acupuncture combined with moxibustion relieves the symptoms of Crohn's disease. Further research is required.

Inform your physician if you use any complementary and alternative medicine. A few of these substances may have an impact on how well drugs or other treatments work. An interaction or side effect may, in certain cases, be dangerous or even life-threatening.

What are the different forms of Crohn's disease?

There are five variations of Crohn's disease, each based on where the illness is located in the digestive system. They are:

Gene-driven dementia with chromosome abnormalities. This rare condition primarily affects you.

Jejunocerebrosis. This type develops in the jejunum, the second portion of your gut. Similar to generic Crohn's disease, this variant is less frequent.

Iledtis.Ilemia involves inflammation in the ileum, the last segment of the small intestine.

Ileocolitis. This is the most prevalent variant of Crohn's disease and affects the colon and ileum.

Crohn's disease. This only affects the coin. Both Crohn's colitis and ulcerative colitis impact the colon superficially; however, Crohn's colitis can also impact the deeper layers of the intestinal lining.

Perianal disease. This frequently involves fistulas, or normal skin surrounding the anus.

Eatables and Avoidables

Grains

Cereals are typical dietary staples. Because whole grains are high in nutrients and fibre, they are frequently used as food and offer the greatest nutritional benefits. According to research, eating a higher-fibre diet may lower your risk of having IBD.

However, after receiving an IBD diagnosis and the disease is active, the fibrillation factor may become problematic. Your doctor may suggest a low-fibre diet according to your symptoms.

This implies that you must restrict the quantity of whole grains you consume. A low-fibre, low-residue diet will help control acute symptoms or minor intestinal constriction. This diet lessens fibre and "scrap" that could linger and aggravate the digestive system.

Nonetheless, continuous research questions the usefulness of low-fiber diets in treating Crohn's disease. A small study conducted in 2015 that used a plant-forward diet that included fish, eggs, dairy, and fibre revealed a high rate of sustained remission over two years.

After reviewing further studies, the researchers concluded that plant-based diets may aid in reducing inflammatory responses and enhancing general health. Researchers reported that the higher fibre intake did not lead to any adverse symptoms or consequences.

Chapter 3: Nutritional Options and Health Benefits

demonstrates research showing vegans naturally have decreased risks for obesity, heart disease, high blood pressure, and several types of cancer when they eat a balanced, low-fat, high-fibre plant-based diet.

Eating a vegan diet typically involves consuming fewer fat and calorie-dense foods such as fruits and vegetables, as opposed to higher-fat meats, dairy products, breads, and cereals.

Saturated Fat Associated with Animals

Unsaturated Fat Associated with Plants

Advantages for Health

Some reasons people become enthusiastic about going vegan include reducing blood pressure and cholesterol, boosting energy, preventing disease, and losing weight. Let's take a closer look at the health advantages.

Heart: High blood pressure, high cholesterol, and heart disease are all associated with excessive saturated fat, which is present in animal products, according to womenshealthmag.com specialists. The leading cause of death for women is heart disease, which can be considerably reduced by adopting a vegan lifestyle.

Research indicates that even a minor decrease in the consumption of this unhealthy fat can enhance heart health.

Cancer: According to the Canadian Cancer Society, red and processed meat eaters are most at risk for the disease. High-fat meats have been linked in numerous studies to pancreatic, liver, prostate, and breast cancers. Going vegan can help lower the risk if you do it healthily.

Reduce Your Weight: Plant-based foods are lower in calories and fat than meat. It indicates that if you eat foods high in fat, such as meat and animal products, your chances of being overweight increase. According to nutritionists, several studies have shown that those who consume meat regularly have a ten-fold higher risk of being overweight compared to vegans. Additionally, meat eaters tend to increase in weight as the years pass.

Put another way, it's safe to assume that choosing a healthy vegan diet will let you lose weight permanently.

Mental Plus: Your thoughts and emotions have. Your perspective on life won't be optimistic if you consume bad food and your head is congested and unhealthy.

According to Psychology Today, having a positive outlook has everything to do with what you eat and how you live, not simply doing what makes you happy. Because of all the simple sugar energy you get from eating a fatty burger and fries, you could feel wonderful for a few minutes afterwards, but it won't take long for you to feel like crap. Your energy and blood sugar levels will decline, leaving you feeling drained and miserable.

A nutritious, low-fat diet will help you feel more energized and turn on a positive outlook. This will positively impact your behaviour, your connections with coworkers, family, and friends, the risks you take and the wise, healthful path you choose to follow in life.

One of the most obvious advantages of adopting a healthy vegan diet is energy. Your energy levels will skyrocket when you feed your body and mind pure, unfiltered, all-natural energy. You'll provide your internal systems sustained energy, stabilize blood sugar, and eliminate the de-energizing mood swings most of us experience during the day. A steady stream of high-quality energy will make you feel amazing from waking up until your head hits the pillow.

Essential Foods for a Vegan Diet

Remember that diversity is essential, and never stop trying out different pairings.

Serving size: 1/4 cup dry fruit or vegetables, cup fresh fruit or vegetables, ten to twelve portions daily

* Bread and Cereals: Steel-cut oats, crackers, rice, and whole wheat bread. Make sure the

grain you are purchasing is whole grain, as this indicates minimal to no processing that removes nutrients. While quick rolled oats aren't the healthiest choice, they are still preferable to white bread!

Serving Size: 1 slice of bread, 5–6 crackers, 3/4 cup cooked cereal, and 3/4 cup rice or pasta

6–8 portions daily

* Soy and Dairy-Free Products: Items like rice milk, coconut milk, almond milk, and soy milk fall under this category. Add to that dairy-free cream cheese, cottage cheese, margarine, and soy yoghurt. Emerg-G Egg Replacer is a vegan egg alternative that is also organic. Seek for all-natural organic items. It seems like more and more plant-based foods are being released every day. Adhere to the recommended serving size and, if possible, select low-fat options.

Serving Size: 1 tbsp, 2 x 2 inch cube of soy cheese, and a vegan egg substitute. 1/2 cup soy ice cream, 3/4 cup soy yoghurt, 1 cup almond milk, and margarine, two to three portions daily

*Seeds, Nuts, and Legumes: Consuming a wide range of these foods is crucial. Nutritious examples include kidney beans, chickpeas, sunflower seeds, lentils, peas, soya beans, walnuts, almonds, cashews, sesame, and flax seeds.

* Serving Size: 3/4 cup kidney beans, 3/4 cup peas, 1/4 cup sunflower seeds, 1/3 cup mixed nuts, 6-8 almonds, two to three portions daily

A vegan diet consists mostly of fresh fruits and vegetables, low in saturated fat, fibre-rich, and healthy complex carbohydrates. If you know how to prepare vegetarian food, it can help you stay in excellent health!

Embracing Life - The Plant-Based Approach

Cracking the Code for a Healthier, Longer Life

A long life becomes a highly sought-after goal in pursuing a fulfilled life. What if the secret to living a longer, healthier life lies not in magical springs or potions but in the ingredients you choose to put on your plate? Start analyzing lifespan from the standpoint of a plant-based lifestyle. This journey goes beyond simple nutrition to sort through the benefits of living off of plants that have been scientifically proven.

Sowing the Seeds of Eternity

Our daily choices, especially those related to our diet, provide the foundation for a long lifespan. A vegan diet emphasizing all plant foods is a powerful tool for achieving a long life. Produce, nuts, beans, and other plant foods are rich in vitamins, minerals, and antioxidants that create a balance of health within your body and fortify it against ageing.

Fighting Off Chronic Illnesses

Chronic illnesses are often very difficult roadblocks to a long and fulfilling life. A vegan diet effectively avoids and reduces several diseases in scientific research. A high-fiber, low-cholesterol, and antioxidant-rich diet can prevent. Adopting a vegan lifestyle allows you to actively combat these adversaries that shorten lives.

Plant-Powered Rejuvenation of Cells

At the cellular level, the results of a vegan diet are a tale of regeneration. Plant compounds that are essential for preserving cellular health include polyphenols and phytochemicals. They serve as defenders, shielding your cells from the two main causes of accelerated ageing—oxidative damage and inflammation. Your cells go through an energetic change that transcends time with the powerful power of plants.

Maintaining Mental Agility

A long life involves caring for your mind, the centre of your existence, and physical health. A vegan diet, rich in antioxidants, brain-protecting compounds, and omega-3 fatty acids, emerges as a mental health champion. According to research, a plant-based diet's anti-inflammatory properties may help reduce the likelihood of cognitive decline and pave the way for a longer, sharper mind.

Improving Life Quality

It's not only about accumulating years; longevity is also about the quality of those years. Living a vegan lifestyle that emphasizes nutrient-dense, complete meals improves your health in general. Join you on your journey to make every day a celebration of living life to the fullest.

A Harmony of Advantages

Finally, veganism creates a harmonious blend of advantages contributing to a longer, healthier life. As you enjoy the variety of tastes of plant-powered nutrition, it becomes clear that this is not just a transient promise but a reality supported by science. As you set out on this adventure, remember that longevity isn't a far-off place; rather, it's a travelling companion who will enhance every step of your colourful, plant-powered voyage.

Bringing Life - The Plant-Based Method for Renewable Energy

Bring Your True Nature Back to Life with Plant-Powered Energy

Finding a reliable power source is crucial in a society where energy is often in short supply. When one embraces a vegan lifestyle, their search for fresh energy and vitality becomes more focused. We will discover the transforming power of plant-based nutrition, bidding farewell to sluggishness and embracing a burst of sustained energy.

Sustaining More Than Calories

Energy is more than just the sum of its calorie counts. The energy and vitality keep our bodies functioning at all levels. Eating veganism prioritizes nutrient-dense meals high in vitamins, minerals, and antioxidants, providing a comprehensive approach to nutrition.

It can give our bodies the vital elements required to perform at their best. Due to their naturally high nutrient content, these foods promote general health and well-being.

Apart from offering an extensive array of nutrients, a vegan diet is frequently obesity and some forms of cancer. It can also help with better digestion and weight management, raising energy levels.

Remember that each person may have different nutritional needs, so it's critical to ensure you eat a well-balanced diet that satisfies them. It can be helpful to work with a qualified dietitian or nutritionist to create a vegan meal plan that meets your needs and guarantees you get all the nutrients you need for maximum energy and vitality.

Whole Foods' Power

Yes, whole foods derived from plants are the foundation for long-term energy. They offer a harmonious blend of nutrients that release energy steadily and gradually.

Our bodies use complex carbohydrates as their main energy source, which can be found in whole grains, legumes, and fruits. Because of their gradual breakdown, blood glucose levels are released steadily into the bloodstream, avoiding sharp rises and falls in energy levels.

Sources of fibre, which helps to sustain energy levels. It prevents blood sugar swings and results in a more consistent release of energy by slowing down glucose absorption.

Important micronutrients found in plant-based diets, such as vitamins and minerals, assist the body's ability to produce energy and maintain general health. B vitamins, for instance, present in leafy greens, legumes, and whole grains, are essential for converting food into energy. On the other hand, creating cell oxygen requires lentils and fortified meals.

On the other hand, refined carbohydrates and processed foods with added sugars can provide you with a brief energy boost, but because blood sugar levels fluctuate quickly, they frequently cause a subsequent crash.

Like the ebb and flow of a life-giving tide, you can experience a calm and consistent energy flow by eating a plant-based diet rich in complete, nutrient-dense foods. It promotes sustained vigour devoid of the transient highs and lows linked to processed diets.

Reducing Energy Wasters

Certain items in non-vegan diets can make you feel drained and sluggish. Saturated fats, animal products, and too much refined sugar deplete your energy.

Avoiding these energy-draining factors can help alleviate these concerns and lead to a vegan lifestyle. A plant-based diet is high in whole grains, legumes, fruits, and vegetables, which provide a variety of minerals and antioxidants to help maintain and increase your energy levels. Furthermore, vegan diets typically contain fewer saturated fats, which might be a factor in sluggishness.

It's crucial to remember that even while a vegan diet might be healthful, making sure you obtain all the nutrients you need is still crucial. Speaking with a nutritionist or dietitian may be beneficial to meet your energy demands while following a vegan diet.

How To Begin Cooking With Pegans

Crucial components in Pegan cuisine

Pegan cooking centres around a few staple foods that align with the diet's goals. These ingredients have been selected for their nutritional value, diversity, and alignment with the Pegan Diet's focus on whole, unprocessed foods. The following are some key ingredients that are frequently used in Pegan cooking:

1. Vegetables and Fruits:

The foundation of Pegan meals is a wide assortment of fruits and vegetables. These consist of cruciferous vegetables, sweet potatoes, berries, avocados, leafy greens, and a variety of vibrant.

2. Nuts and Seeds: Nuts and seeds provide essential nutrients, protein, and healthy fats. These include almonds, walnuts, chia seeds, flaxseeds, and pumpkin seeds. They are adaptable ingredients that add flavour, texture, and nutrition to Pegan cuisine.

3. Lean Proteins: An essential component of Pegan cooking is high-quality, lean proteins derived from animals such as wild-caught fish, pasture-raised poultry, grass-fed cattle, and plant-based substitutes like tempeh and tofu. These proteins meet vegan and paleo dietary standards and ensure a well-balanced macronutrient composition.

4. Healthy Fats: Nutritious fatty acids are found in foods like avocados, almonds, coconut oil, and olive oil. Healthy fats are a major component of Pegan's cooking. These fats improve the nutritional profile of Pegan meals overall, provide satiety, and promote brain function.

5. Gluten-Free Grains: Quinoa, brown rice, and millet are gluten-free grains frequently used in vegan recipes. These grains support the diet's emphasis on whole, minimally processed foods by serving as a source of fibre, additional nutrients, and complex carbohydrates.

6. Plant-Based Proteins: In vegan cooking, legumes, lentils, and beans are important sources of plant-based proteins. These foods contribute to the balanced approach of the diet by providing a high-protein profile, fibre, and many minerals.

7. Herbs and Spices: Without using a lot of sugar or salt, herbs and spices are utilised to

improve the flavours of Pegan cuisine. Common choices include garlic, turmeric, cumin, mint, cilantro, basil, and cumin, which provide variety and depth to the culinary experience.

8. Non-Dairy replacements: Almond milk, coconut milk, and cashew cheese are examples of non-dairy replacements frequently used in vegan cooking. These substitutes offer choices for creamy textures and flavours while still adhering to the diet's restriction on dairy.

9. Fermented Foods: By providing advantageous probiotics, fermented foods like kimchi, kombucha, and sauerkraut improve gut health. Including these aligns with the holistic approach to health that the Pegan Diet takes.

10. Low-Glycemic Sweeteners: Pegan recipes can incorporate low-glycemic sweeteners like monk fruit, coconut sugar, or maple syrup when sweetness is needed. These options help control blood sugar levels in line with the diet's guidelines.

By including these essential components in Pegan cooking, users may create various delicious, well-balanced meals that align with the diet's primary health and sustainability goals.

OVERVIEW

I thought of you right away and wanted to take a moment to acknowledge the significant impact that "The Skinnytaste Simple Cookbook" has made on my culinary journey. This cookbook is so much more than that; it's a culinary manual that has changed how I think about food and cooking.

I was swept up in a world of intriguing and familiar flavours from the first recipe. Your book is a constant companion, teaching me how to make tasty meals on a tight budget without sacrificing flavour.

Maria, your well-considered advice and simple-to-follow recipe books have improved my culinary abilities and brought happiness and inspiration into my kitchen. Your focus on keeping things simple and honouring inexpensive components has changed the game.

The way your cookbook has inspired inventiveness with leftovers is among its most impressive features. I used to think leftovers were boring, but after seeing your creative transformations, I now see many more possibilities. I am very grateful to you for making every meal seem like it has been revitalised.

My relationship with food has significantly transformed thanks to your enthusiasm and knowledge. I've learned from your cookbook that all it takes is a little Skinnytaste magic to create a tasty, nutritious meal without breaking the pocketbook.

What strikes a chord with me the most goes beyond the delectable recipes: the emotion you've infused into each page. It's about creating moments, memories, and a sense of community—it's not just about cooking. Your comments have a special way of bringing warmth and love into my kitchen, making it a creative and loving space.

Maria, I appreciate you sharing your cooking knowledge and writing an exceptional cookbook. I deeply appreciate your commitment to sharing the joy of easy, affordable meals with others, as it has profoundly affected my life.

Yummy Vegan Chronosomic Cookbook

1. Quinoa Power Bowl

Ingredients:

- 1 cup cherry tomatoes, halved
- 1/2 cup shredded carrots

- 1/4 cup chopped fresh cilantro
- 1 cup quinoa
- 2 cups water
- 1 cup diced cucumber

Preparation:

1. Wash the quinoa in cool water.
2. For fifteen minutes, simmer, cover, and reduce heat.
3. Once the quinoa is fluffy, let it cool.
4. Combine the quinoa, veggies, and cilantro in a bowl.

CRISPY Baked ZUCCHINI FRIES

PREP TIME: 15 MINUTES**COOK TIME**: 25 MINUTES

SERVINGS: 4 PORTIONS

NUTRITIONAL BREAKDOWN (PER SERVING):

CALORIES: **90**
PROTEIN: **5G**
CARBOHYDRATES: **18G**
FAT: 1G
FIBER: **3G**

INGREDIENTS:

- 1/2 teaspoon paprika
- Salt and pepper to taste
- Cooking spray
- 2 medium zucchinis
- 1/2 cup breadcrumbs
- 1/4 cup nutritional yeast
- 1 teaspoon garlic powder

INSTRUCTIONS:

1. Adjust the oven temperature to 425°F (220°) pan.

2. Cut zucchini into sticks that resemble fries.
3. Combine breadcrumbs, nutritional yeast, paprika, garlic powder, salt, and pepper in a bowl.
4. Coat the zucchini sticks with the mixture of breadcrumbs.
5. Coat them with cooking spray after putting them on the baking sheet.
6. Until crisp and golden.
7. If preferred, serve with a dipping sauce.

www.ingramcontent.com/pod-product-compliance
Lightning Source LLC
Chambersburg PA
CBHW070031040426
42333CB00040B/1428